THE ART AND S AURICULOT

CW00508051

A Comprehensive Analysis Of The Life-Changing Effects Of Auriculotherapy

JENSEN DAVID

Contents

CHAPTER ONE
Auriculotherapy: An Overview

Auriculotherapy is a form of alternative medicine that involves stimulating certain sites on the outer ear to improve health and well-being. It is also known as ear acupuncture or ear reflexology. Auriculotherapy has been practiced for thousands of years in many different cultures all over the world, including but not limited to China, Egypt, and Greece.

Auriculotherapy is predicated on the idea that the ear is a miniature version of the rest of the body, with corresponding reaction sites and acupuncture meridians. It is claimed that the corresponding organs or systems in the body can be altered and balanced by stimulating these points using various techniques, such as pressure, needles, or electrical stimulation.

Pain management, stress reduction, addiction treatment, digestive difficulties, and emotional well-being are just some of the many conditions for which auriculotherapy is utilized as a complimentary or adjunct therapy.

It is a gentle and non-invasive treatment option that can stand on its own or complement other therapies.

A qualified practitioner who is familiar with ear anatomy and the locations that correspond to other parts of the body is most suited to administer auriculotherapy. Treatment programs are generally tailored to the individual needs of each patient and may require multiple visits before any noticeable improvement is shown.

Although many people have experienced success with

auriculotherapy, there is a lack of robust scientific data to support its use at this time. If you have any preexisting health disorders or concerns, you should talk to your doctor before considering auriculotherapy or any other alternative treatment.

Concepts And Ideas At The Ground Level

Several fundamental ideas and principles underpin the practice of auriculotherapy. For example:

• Based on the idea that the ear represents a miniature version of the body's various systems and that acupuncture sites on the ear are directly related to those in the rest of the body, auriculotherapy treats a wide range of conditions. It is hypothesized that a web of nerve fibers and energy channels connects all of these nodes.

• Auriculotherapy is related to reflexology, a technique whereby pressure is applied to specific locations on the hands, feet, or ears in order to activate the corresponding parts of the body.

Stimulating these spots is said to improve both physical and mental health; practices like auriculotherapy and reflexology take this premise as their starting point.

• Notions from Traditional Chinese Medicine (TCM) Auriculotherapy is based on TCM notions including yin and yang, meridians, and qi (vital life force energy). Traditional Chinese Medicine (TCM) holds that activating acupoints on the ear can improve health by reestablishing internal yin and yang harmony, qi flow, and overall wellbeing.

• Auriculotherapy is often adapted to meet the specific requirements of each particular patient. Because everyone's ears are different, the acupressure spots used to treat a certain illness or symptom may change from patient to patient. A qualified practitioner will evaluate the patient's health, consider the patient's medical history, and determine which ear points are most appropriate for the patient's treatment.

• Auriculotherapy can be performed with a variety of methods, such as physical pressure, acupuncture needles, electrical stimulation, magnets, or ear-attached seeds or tapes. The patient's preferences, the nature of the ailment, and the practitioner's skill set are all potential factors in determining the approach taken.

• Auriculotherapy is commonly utilized as a complimentary or adjunct therapy, meaning it is used in conjunction with primary care, mainstream medicine, and alternative medicine.

It is not supposed to take the place of regular medical attention, but rather work in tandem with it to improve health and wellness.

• Auriculotherapy is holistic since it treats the whole person, including the mind, body, and spirit. It recognizes the interconnectedness of the body and aims to treat the underlying causes of illness rather than just the symptoms.

If you have any preexisting health conditions or concerns, it is essential that you discuss auriculotherapy with a trained medical expert before to beginning treatment.

CHAPTER TWO
Auriculotherapy's Pros And Cons

The potential advantages and disadvantages of auriculotherapy are similar to those of any other therapeutic method. Some pros and cons of auriculotherapy are as follows.

Auriculotherapy's Pluses

• Auriculotherapy is widely regarded as a safe and non-invasive treatment option. Some people who prefer more natural and holistic approaches to health may appreciate that it does not require the use of pharmaceuticals or invasive procedures.

• Auriculotherapy may be useful for pain relief, and it has been used successfully to treat chronic pain problems like arthritis, back pain, and migraines. Stimulating acupoints on the ear is thought to cause the body to produce endorphins, which are hormones that reduce pain.

• Auriculotherapy has been utilized as an alternative method of treating stress and anxiety. Stimulating specific auricular sites is thought to restore the body's energy flow and foster feelings of peace and serenity.

• Auriculotherapy is often adapted to the specific needs of each patient, with individualized treatment regimens developed in light of each person's condition, symptoms, and reaction to treatment. Some people, especially those who value individuality and holistic medicine, could appreciate this bespoke approach.

• Auriculotherapy can be used in conjunction with traditional medicine or other alternative therapies for a more holistic approach.

It can be used in conjunction with other therapeutic techniques and as part of a bigger treatment plan to promote health and wellness.

Auriculotherapy's Downsides:

• Although many auriculotherapists and their patients have reported excellent results from using this technique, the scientific evidence supporting its use is still scant and contradictory. To prove its usefulness for a wide range of ailments, more rigorous study is required.

• Knowledgeable practitioners are needed for auriculotherapy because of the complexity of the ear's architecture, the location of reflex points, and the specificity of the treatments required. The efficacy of treatment may vary depending on the practitioner's experience and education.

• As with any therapeutic method, some people may respond better to auriculotherapy than others. It is possible that some people will see major improvements, while others will not react at all or will only see little ones.

• Auriculotherapy is not intended to be used alone, but rather as a supplement to standard medical treatment. Never attempt to diagnose or treat a medical problem without first speaking with a trained medical practitioner; this includes even minor ailments.

• Even though auriculotherapy has a low risk of adverse effects, there is still a chance of infection, bruising, or discomfort because of the use of needles or electrical stimulation.

Prior to receiving treatment, you should check that the practitioner is following all necessary safety precautions and hygiene standards.

• Auriculotherapy is not for everyone since it could not be safe for people with certain health issues, allergies, or sensitivities. If you have any preexisting health conditions or concerns, it is essential that you discuss auriculotherapy with a trained medical expert before to beginning treatment.

Auriculotherapy, like any other alternative treatment, should be approached with skepticism and knowledge.

If you have any preexisting health ailments or concerns, you should talk to a doctor before considering auriculotherapy or any other alternative treatment.

CHAPTER THREE
The Ear: Its Structure And Function

The ear is a multi-functional organ that helps us hear and keep our equilibrium. The ear consists of the external ear, the middle ear, and the central auditory system.

• The outer ear is the easily seen region of the ear responsible for gathering sound waves and channeling them into the ear canal. The external ear consists of the pinna and the ear canal, a tube-like structure that connects the pinna to the middle ear.

• The eardrum (tympanic membrane) and the ossicles (malleus, incus, and stapes) are found in the middle ear, which is situated between the outer and inner ears.

When sound waves strike the eardrum, they cause it to vibrate, and those vibrations are carried via the ossicles to the inner ear.

• The inner ear processes sound by transforming it into electrical impulses for transmission to the brain. It is also vital to maintaining equilibrium. The semicircular canals, the vestibule, and the cochlea are all parts of the inner ear.

The hair cells in the cochlea are crucial for hearing, and they send electrical signals up the auditory nerve to the brain. The vestibule and semicircular canals help us maintain our equilibrium by picking up on shifts in head position and movement.

An intricate system of blood arteries, nerves, and muscles all contribute to the ear's overall function.

The auditory system relies on blood vessels for oxygen and nutrients, and the auditory nerve for signal transmission to the brain. Ear muscles aid in sound localisation and regulating eardrum tension for the best possible hearing.

Auriculotherapy relies on stimulating specific locations on the ear to alter various physiological processes and encourage healing, therefore familiarity with ear anatomy and physiology is helpful.

Auriculotherapy is based on and relies heavily on the ear's complex anatomy and network of nerves, muscles, and organs.

Methods And Equipment For Auriculotherapy

Auriculotherapy is the practice of applying pressure to a series of acupressure points on the outer ear in an effort to treat and prevent health issues. In auriculotherapy, these sites are stimulated using a variety of equipment and methods. These are some of the most typical methods and equipment:

• In order to find and stimulate certain areas on the ear, a small, pointed instrument called an auricular probe is employed. Usually constructed of stainless steel, its rounded tip gently stimulates acupressure points in the ear.

In order to elicit a reaction from the ear, the auricular probe is used to palpate the area and apply pressure or light mechanical stimulation.

• Small, adhesive seeds or pellets composed of metal or other materials are put to precise spots on the ear and left there for continual stimulation; this technique is known as "ear seeding" or "ear pelleting." They are a covert and inconspicuous option for long-term auricular (ear) point stimulation.

• The ear locations can be stimulated with a mild electrical current using a technique called electrical stimulation. Auriculotherapy devices can be used to target specific areas of the ear with mild electrical stimulation. Stimulating the auricular sites with electricity is thought to increase the therapy's effectiveness.

• In laser stimulation, low-level laser therapy is used to activate acupoints in the ear in a noninvasive manner. When a low-powered laser is directed at certain places on the ear, the absorbed energy stimulates tissue repair and reduces pain.

• Applying pressure, rubbing, or kneading certain places on the ear is what massage and pressure treatments are all about. These methods have been shown to be effective in stimulating the spots, soothing the ear muscles, and facilitating healing.

• The process of applying heat to the ear locations is known as thermal stimulation. Several techniques exist for this purpose, including the application of heat in the form of warm compresses, heated probes, or moxibustion (the localized burning of a herb called mugwort around the ear points).

The practitioner's background, the patient's health, and the therapist's personal preferences can all influence the methods and equipment employed in auriculotherapy. In order to provide safe and effective treatment, auriculotherapists must be well-versed in the principles of the practice and possess the necessary training and equipment.

CHAPTER FOUR
Explaining The Various Ear Points And What They Do In Great Detail

Auriculotherapy is the practice of applying pressure to a series of acupressure points on the outer ear in an effort to treat and prevent health issues.

Stimulating these spots can initiate a response that aids in reestablishing equilibrium and promoting wellness because they are thought to be linked to many organs, systems, and activities of the body via neural pathways. Listed below are some of the most often visited auricular treatment ear sites and the associated functions:

• Shen Men (Spirit Gate) is a "master point" in auriculotherapy and is used for general relaxation, stress reduction, and emotional well-being. It may be found at the top of the ear, in the triangular fossa. It has been said to help with sleeplessness, sadness, and anxiety.

• The center of the earlobe, known as Point Zero, is a balancing point that is utilized to encourage homeostasis and restore equilibrium. It has been used to treat a wide variety of health problems and is thought to have a balancing impact on the body as a whole.

• Asthma, cough, and respiratory infections are among illnesses connected with the respiratory system that are typically treated by stimulating the Lung Point, which is located on the upper half of the antitragus. It is thought that by stimulating this location, respiratory symptoms can be alleviated and lung function can be enhanced.

• The Kidney Point is a common acupuncture point for treating kidney problems, back pain, and erectile dysfunction because of its proximity to the urinary and reproductive systems. It is commonly thought to strengthen the kidneys and encourage regular urination and conception.

• The Liver Point, found in the middle of the antitragus, is a popular acupuncture site for treating liver diseases, as well as for detoxifying and menstruation problems. It is believed that stimulating this point will aid in liver health, detoxification, and menstrual cycle control.

• The Digestive Point is a popular acupuncture site for treating digestive-related issues like indigestion, nausea, and gastrointestinal diseases. It is located at the bottom edge of the earlobe. It is thought that by stimulating this spot, both digestion and digestive symptoms might be improved.

• The endocrine system consists of glands like the pituitary, thyroid, and adrenals; the Endocrine Point is located on the inner half of the antitragus and corresponds to this system.

It is frequently prescribed for cases of hormonal discord, metabolic ailment, and stress-related illness. Stimulating this acupoint is said to have a balancing effect on hormones and the endocrine system.

• Acupuncture sites on the ear can be utilized to alleviate a variety of aches and pains, including those in the head, neck, back, and joints. Auriculotherapy is the practice of stimulating these auricular sites to alleviate pain and other symptoms.

It is vital to keep in mind that different auriculotherapy systems may have somewhat different mappings or interpretations of the ear points, which could lead to some minor differences in where and how they are used.

Accurately locating and stimulating the ear spots is crucial to the success of auriculotherapy, but this can only be done with the proper training and understanding of the principles involved.

Auriculotherapy For Various Physical Illnesses

Stimulating auricular (ear) points can be utilized as an adjunct to conventional medicine for a number of physical health issues.

Stimulating these ear spots may assist restore equilibrium and promote healing since they are thought to be linked to various organs, systems, and activities of the body via neural connections. Some physical health issues that may benefit from auriculotherapy include the following:

• Auriculotherapy is commonly used for pain management since it is thought that specific sites on the ear correspond to specific pain centers throughout the body.

Acupressure, acupuncture, and microcurrent stimulation are only few of the methods that have been shown to be effective in relieving the pain and discomfort caused by illnesses including headaches, migraines, musculoskeletal pain, and neuropathic pain by stimulating these sites.

• Indigestion, bloating, constipation, diarrhea, and irritable bowel syndrome (IBS) are just some of the digestive issues that auriculotherapy can help with.

Stimulating ear points related to the digestive system has been shown to aid digestion, normalize bowel motions, and reduce gastrointestinal discomfort.

• Asthma, allergies, cough, and sinus congestion are just some of the respiratory ailments that auriculotherapy might aid in treating. Stimulating ear points related to the respiratory system can enhance lung function, decrease inflammation, and alleviate respiratory symptoms.

• Migraines, headaches, neuropathies, and multiple sclerosis are all neurological diseases that may benefit from the addition of auriculotherapy to standard care.

Some people feel that stimulating a few spots on the ear can aid with nerve regulation, inflammation reduction, and the alleviation of neurological symptoms.

• Auriculotherapy is useful for treating hormonal imbalances and its related symptoms, including

PMS, hot flashes, and irritability during menopause. Stimulating acupoints on the ear that are linked to the endocrine system can improve hormonal balance and reduce associated symptoms.

• Insomnia, RLS, and Sleep Apnea are just few of the sleep disorders that auriculotherapy has been shown to help with. Stimulating specific auricular points has been shown to improve the quantity and quality of sleep by lowering tension and promoting relaxation.

• Auriculotherapy has been utilized as a complementary treatment for nicotine, alcohol, and opiate withdrawal, among others.

Stimulating ear points related to addiction and detoxification has been shown to lessen drug use and its accompanying cravings and withdrawal symptoms.

A certified healthcare expert who is trained in auriculotherapy should provide the treatment, and auriculotherapy should be utilized as a complimentary therapy in addition to traditional medical care.

Proper assessment, diagnosis, and treatment planning should be performed by a trained professional, as the specific points, procedures, and protocols may differ based on the individual and the condition being treated.

CHAPTER FIVE
Auriculotherapy As A Treatment For Emotional And Mental Distress

Stimulating acupoints in the outer ear, a procedure known as auriculotherapy, has been used to treat physical ailments for centuries.

Stimulating specific spots on the ear is said to have a positive effect on emotional health by balancing hormones, lowering stress, and improving overall mood. For your mental and emotional well-being, consider these applications of auriculotherapy:

• Anxiety and Stress: Auriculotherapy can be used to alleviate both by stimulating a series of auricular sites known to elicit a calming effect. Stress and anxiety can be alleviated by the use of techniques like acupressure, acupuncture, and microcurrent stimulation, which target these sites.

• Auriculotherapy can be used as an adjunctive treatment for depression and other mood disorders. Stimulating the amygdala and hippocampus, two ear points linked to mood control, has been shown to normalize neurotransmitter levels in the brain, boost mood, and reduce depressive symptoms.

- Post-traumatic stress disorder (PTSD) and other trauma-related illnesses may benefit from auriculotherapy as part of a holistic treatment approach. Stimulating specific auricular points can assist control emotional reactions, lessen the impact of traumatic memories, and promote emotional recovery. These points correspond to the prefrontal cortex and the limbic system, which are involved in the processing of these memories.

• Addiction and emotional eating are linked to a person's emotional state, making auriculotherapy a useful complementary treatment. Stimulating specific auricular points has been shown to aid in the management of emotional triggers, the suppression of cravings, and the maintenance of sobriety from addictive behaviors.

• Auriculotherapy can be used to treat insomnia and other sleep disorders, and to encourage the regular, restful sleep that is so important to physical and mental health.

Stimulating ear points for relaxation and sleep regulation has been shown to increase the quality of sleep, decrease instances of insomnia, and foster a sense of emotional stability.

• Ailments Caused by Stress: Auriculotherapy is effective for treating stress-related ailments such headaches, stomachaches, and migraines. Stimulating ear points for stress relief, relaxation, and emotional equilibrium can aid with stress management and general emotional health.

- Auriculotherapy can be used to promote emotional well-being and resilience through the process of general emotional balancing. Emotional wellness, stress relief, and balance can all be improved by stimulating ear points linked to the hypothalamus and pituitary gland.

A certified healthcare expert educated in auriculotherapy should deliver the treatment, and auriculotherapy should be utilized as a complimentary therapy in addition to standard mental health care.

Proper assessment, diagnosis, and treatment planning should be performed by a trained professional, as the specific points, procedures, and protocols may differ based on the individual and the condition being treated.

Targeted Auricular Therapy For Vulnerable Groups

Infants, children, expectant mothers, and the elderly are just some of the groups that can benefit from auriculotherapy's complementary therapeutic approach. Some things to keep in mind while employing auriculotherapy on specific groups:

• Auriculotherapy has been shown to be effective in treating a variety of health problems in infants and children, including colic, sleep disruptions, respiratory issues, and behavioral abnormalities.

Children and newborns, however, require extra caution because of the vulnerability of their hearing. Treatment for children should be gentler and shorter than for adults, using techniques such as finger pressure or non-invasive approaches like microcurrent stimulation.

Seeds or magnets, which are smaller and less invasive, may also be preferred in pediatric auriculotherapy.

• Pregnant women can utilize auriculotherapy for relief from nausea and vomiting, discomfort, anxiety, and sleeplessness. It is important to take precautions and utilize gentle methods during pregnancy.

Unless otherwise directed by a skilled healthcare expert educated in auriculotherapy, certain sites on the ear, including those linked with reproductive organs, should be avoided during pregnancy.

• Auriculotherapy is useful for the treatment of a variety of symptoms experienced by the elderly, including pain, sleep difficulties, gastrointestinal issues, and cognitive loss.

However, the individual's current health condition, past medical history, and current pharmaceutical regimen must all be taken into account. The treatment should be administered gently, and it should be adjusted based on the patient's responses.

• People with Disabilities Auriculotherapy can be used to treat a wide range of medical disorders, including those related to the mind and body, in people with disabilities.

However, extra measures should be made to guarantee the well-being of those with disabilities throughout the course of their therapy. The treatment process should be explained using communication strategies appropriate for the individual's needs, and the methods and resources employed should be adapted to the patient's strengths and weaknesses.

- People with Diabetes, Hypertension, and Autoimmune Disorders: Auriculotherapy can be used as a supplemental therapy for people with these problems to alleviate symptoms and improve their health and well-being.

However, appropriate assessment and monitoring must be performed, and the treatment plan must be adapted to each patient's unique health status and requirements.

A certified healthcare provider who is knowledgeable about the needs and considerations of unique populations and has received training in auriculotherapy should always perform auriculotherapy. To ensure the safe and effective use of auriculotherapy in unique populations, accurate assessment, diagnosis, and treatment planning are required.

CHAPTER SIX
Clinical Application Of Auriculotherapy

To use auriculotherapy in clinical settings, it must be used as an adjunct to standard medical care. Incorporating auriculotherapy into clinical practice necessitates paying attention to the following details:

• Pre-Auriculotherapy Patient Assessment Collecting the patient's medical history, current health status, and any contraindications or precautions is essential before beginning auriculotherapy. This evaluation should occur in tandem with the patient's standard medical care, and the auriculotherapy treatment plan should be created specifically for the patient.

• The results of the evaluation should inform the creation of a treatment strategy tailored to the individual patient's needs. Planned aspects of auricular therapy may include point selection, treatment methodology, and schedule.

Each patient's treatment plan should be evaluated on a regular basis to ensure it is meeting their needs.

• Auriculotherapy is most effective when it is part of a comprehensive treatment plan developed in collaboration with the patient's other healthcare providers.

A more comprehensive and coordinated approach to patient treatment can be achieved by collaboration and communication with other healthcare providers such as physicians, nurses, and practitioners of complementary and alternative medicine.

• The medical record should include detailed documentation of all auriculotherapy sessions. This involves keeping track of the auricular points treated, the methods and equipment employed, the patient's response to treatment, and any untoward or unexpected outcomes witnessed.

Keeping detailed records allows medical staff to better coordinate care and monitor patient outcomes.

• Patients should be made aware of the possible benefits of auriculotherapy and its role as a supplementary therapy. Limitations of auriculotherapy, projected results, and risks/side effects should all be covered in patient education.

Patients should be encouraged to take an active role in their care and to keep their healthcare providers updated on any changes or concerns they may have.

• Auriculotherapy should be performed using standard precautions for preventing the spread of infection. Hygiene is essential, as is the use of sterile or disposable equipment. Any signs of illness or allergy should be reported to your doctor right away.

• Professional Development and Continuing Education: Healthcare providers should keep abreast of the newest findings in auriculotherapy research. This aids in ensuring that the most up-to-date, evidence-based methods are used in the practice of auriculotherapy.

A full knowledge of auriculotherapy, appropriate assessment and treatment planning, coordination with the healthcare team, documentation, patient education, safety precautions, and ongoing education are all necessary for successful integration into clinical practice. Providers can deliver a more integrative and person-centered approach to health and wellness when they include auriculotherapy as part of their standard practice.

Auriculotherapy: Ethical And Safety Considerations

Auriculotherapy practitioners, like those in any healthcare field, have a responsibility to put patient welfare first and operate ethically at all times. Important issues of ethics and safety to keep in mind when performing auriculotherapy are as follows.

• Patients should give their informed consent for auriculotherapy before any treatment begins. All available options and alternatives must be discussed, as well as the nature of the treatment, any dangers involved, and the anticipated results.

The right to ask questions and make educated decisions regarding one's care is a basic human right.

• Practitioners of auriculotherapy owe a duty of confidentiality to their patients and should treat their information securely in accordance with the law. The medical history, treatment data, and other personal information of patients should be kept private and not shared without their permission.

• Auriculotherapists should exercise expertise in their field and stay within the boundaries of their legal authority when treating patients.

Auriculotherapists should only treat patients for diseases within their area of expertise and refer those with more serious issues to other skilled medical professionals.

• For the sake of their patients, auriculotherapists should take all necessary precautions to prevent the spread of infection. Using sterile or single-use equipment, keeping clean, and following standard protocol are all part of infection control. Any infections or allergic reactions must be treated immediately.

• Auriculotherapists should always act in a professional manner when interacting with patients, coworkers, and other medical personnel. Some examples of this are setting healthy boundaries, treating patients with compassion and respect, and acting with honesty and integrity at all times.

• Treatments for auriculotherapy should be based on the most up-to-date evidence, and practitioners should not exaggerate or misrepresent the therapy's benefits. They need to keep up with the latest findings in the area and evaluate the strength of the evidence for auriculotherapy's efficacy.

• Practitioners of auriculotherapy should be polite and sensitive to the cultural backgrounds of their patients. When formulating plans of care and communicating with patients, healthcare providers should take into account the patients' cultural norms and values as much as possible.

• Respect for and encouragement of patient independence are essential tenets of auriculotherapy.

Respecting patients' autonomy requires listening to their input, giving them information, and letting them choose their own course of treatment.

• Auriculotherapists who want to be at the top of their game should make time for regular sessions of continuing education and other forms of professional development.

To maintain a safe and effective practice, auriculotherapists should keep up with the latest findings in the field.

Practitioners of auriculotherapy can better serve their patients and advance the field's expertise and reputation by following established ethical principles and placing a premium on patient safety.

Conclusion

When it comes to diagnosing and treating a wide variety of physical, mental, and emotional health disorders, auriculotherapy is one of the most novel and successful forms of complementary and alternative medicine.

It was developed from TCM principles and has been used for centuries across cultural boundaries.

In this book, we have covered the fundamentals of auriculotherapy, including its origins, the ear's anatomy and physiology, the methods and techniques used in practice, the most frequently used ear points and their effects, and its applications for a variety of physical health issues, psychological issues, and special populations.

We have also emphasized the significance of ethical and safety considerations in auriculotherapy, including the following: obtaining informed consent, keeping patient information confidential, working within one's area of expertise, taking all necessary precautions to protect patients, acting professionally at all times, basing treatment decisions on scientific evidence, being sensitive to patients' cultural backgrounds, honoring patients' right to make their own treatment decisions, and participating in ongoing training.

Integrating auriculotherapy into clinical practice has been shown to be an effective supplementary therapy to standard medical care. Auriculotherapists should, nevertheless, be professional, follow applicable ethical standards, and put patient well-being first.

Delivering safe and effective care to patients requires an interdisciplinary approach, regular communication with other healthcare professionals, and a commitment to using the best available evidence in clinical practice.

Auriculotherapy, in conclusion, takes into account the interdependence of the body, mind, and spirit to promote health and wellness.

It is a low-risk, low-cost treatment option that can stand on its own or be combined with more traditional or alternative methods. Auriculotherapy has the potential to be an invaluable addition to healthcare practice if practitioners are well trained, knowledgeable, and ethically grounded to do so.

THE END

Printed in Great Britain
by Amazon

27453177R00046